The DASH Diet Cookbook

Easy, Delicious and Healthy Recipes to Lower Blood Pressure

Nelson Lucas

CHAPTER ONE

INTRODUCTION TO THE DASH DIET

What is the DASH diet?

The DASH diet is a dietary pattern designed to help lower blood pressure and reduce the risk of heart disease. DASH stands for Dietary Approaches to Stop Hypertension, and it was developed by the National Heart, Lung, and Blood Institute (NHLBI) as a result of extensive research.

The DASH diet emphasizes eating whole, minimally processed foods and limits high-fat, high-sugar, and high-sodium foods. It encourages eating plenty of fruits, vegetables, whole grains, lean protein sources, and low-fat dairy products. The DASH diet is rich in important nutrients such as fiber, potassium, calcium, and magnesium.

Studies have shown that following the DASH diet can lead to significant reductions in blood pressure, which is a major risk factor for heart disease.

The diet has also been associated with other health benefits, including improved cholesterol levels, better insulin sensitivity, and reduced risk of stroke and certain cancers.

The DASH diet is a flexible and balanced approach to eating that can be adapted to meet individual needs and preferences. It can be a helpful tool for anyone looking to improve their overall health and reduce their risk of chronic diseases.

The history of the DASH diet

The DASH diet was developed in the 1990s by researchers at the National Heart, Lung, and Blood Institute (NHLBI), which is part of the National Institutes of Health (NIH). The NHLBI was looking for ways to reduce high blood pressure, which is a major risk factor for heart disease and stroke.

The NHLBI conducted a series of clinical trials to study the effects of dietary patterns on blood pressure. These trials involved over 450 participants and were conducted over the course of several years.

The first clinical trial, called the DASH-Sodium trial, was conducted from 1994 to 1995. The trial compared the effects of three different diets on blood pressure: a typical

American diet, a diet rich in fruits and vegetables, and the DASH diet, which was designed to be rich in fruits, vegetables, whole grains, lean protein, and low-fat dairy.

The results of the DASH-Sodium trial showed that the DASH diet was the most effective at lowering blood pressure, particularly when combined with a reduced sodium intake.

Subsequent trials confirmed these findings and showed that the DASH diet could also improve cholesterol levels, reduce the risk of stroke, and lower the risk of developing heart disease.

Today, the DASH diet is widely recommended as a healthy eating pattern for everyone, not just those with high blood pressure.

It has been recognized by numerous organizations, including the American Heart Association, as an effective way to reduce the risk of heart disease and other chronic illnesses.

The principles of the DASH diet

The DASH diet is based on several principles, which include:

Emphasizing whole, minimally processed foods:
The DASH diet encourages eating plenty of fruits, vegetables, whole grains, lean protein sources, and low-fat dairy products. These foods are rich in important nutrients such as fiber, potassium, calcium, and magnesium.

Limiting high-fat, high-sugar, and high-sodium foods:
The DASH diet restricts foods that are high in saturated and trans fats, added sugars, and sodium. These foods can contribute to high blood pressure, high cholesterol levels, and other health problems.

Increasing potassium intake: Potassium is an important nutrient that can help lower blood pressure.

The DASH diet recommends eating potassium-rich foods such as fruits, vegetables, beans, and low-fat dairy products.

Reducing sodium intake: Sodium is a mineral that can raise blood pressure. The DASH diet recommends limiting sodium intake to 2,300 milligrams per day, or even less for those with high blood pressure or other health conditions.

Balancing macronutrients: The DASH diet emphasizes a balance of carbohydrates, protein, and healthy fats. It recommends getting most of your calories from carbohydrates, particularly from whole grains, and limiting saturated and trans fats.

Adapting to individual needs: The DASH diet is a flexible and adaptable approach to eating. It can be adjusted to meet individual needs and preferences, while still following the basic principles of the diet

The health benefits of the DASH diet

The DASH diet has been shown to have numerous health benefits, including:

Lowering blood pressure: Studies have consistently shown that the DASH diet can help lower blood pressure in people with high blood pressure. It has also been shown to prevent high blood pressure from developing in people with normal blood pressure.

Reducing the risk of heart disease: The DASH diet has been associated with a reduced risk of developing heart disease, including heart attacks, heart failure, and stroke. This is likely due to the diet's emphasis on whole, minimally processed foods and its restriction of high-fat, high-sugar, and high-sodium foods.

Improving cholesterol levels: The DASH diet has been shown to improve cholesterol levels by reducing levels of LDL ("bad") cholesterol and increasing levels of HDL ("good") cholesterol.

Lowering the risk of diabetes: The DASH diet has been associated with a reduced risk of developing type 2 diabetes. This is likely due to the diet's emphasis on whole grains, fruits, vegetables, and lean protein sources, which can help regulate blood sugar levels.

Improving overall health: The DASH diet is a balanced and nutrient-dense eating pattern that can improve overall health and well-being. It is rich in important nutrients such as fiber, potassium, calcium, and magnesium, and can help reduce the risk of chronic diseases such as cancer, osteoporosis, and kidney disease.

Overall, the DASH diet is a healthy and sustainable approach to eating that can have numerous health benefits for people of all ages and backgrounds.

CHAPTER TWO
THE IMPORTANCE OF NUTRITION

The role of macronutrients in the diet

Macronutrients are the three main nutrients that the body needs in large amounts to function properly: carbohydrates, protein, and fat.

The role of each macronutrient in the diet is as follows:

Carbohydrates:

Carbohydrates are the body's primary source of energy. They are broken down into glucose, which is used by the body for fuel. The DASH diet emphasizes complex carbohydrates, such as whole grains, fruits, and vegetables, which provide sustained energy and important nutrients such as fiber, vitamins, and minerals.

Protein:

Protein is essential for building and repairing tissues in the body, including muscles, bones, and organs. The DASH diet emphasizes lean protein sources, such as fish, poultry, beans, and nuts, which are lower in saturated fat and higher in important nutrients such as omega-3 fatty acids and fiber.

Fat:

Fat is essential for many bodily functions, including hormone production, vitamin absorption, and insulation. The DASH diet emphasizes healthy fats, such as those found in nuts, seeds, avocados, and olive oil, which can help reduce inflammation and lower the risk of heart disease.

It is important to note that the DASH diet does not restrict any particular macronutrient, but rather emphasizes a balance of all three.

The diet recommends getting most of your calories from carbohydrates, but also includes lean protein sources and healthy fats in moderate amounts.
A balanced macronutrient intake can help provide the body with the energy and nutrients it needs to function properly and maintain optimal health.

Importance of Micronutrients

Micronutrients are essential nutrients that the body needs in small amounts to function properly, including vitamins and minerals.

While they are needed in smaller quantities than macronutrients, they play important roles in the body, such as:

Supporting immune function:

Many micronutrients, such as vitamins C, D, and E, and zinc, play important roles in supporting immune function and helping the body fight off infections and illnesses.

Maintaining healthy bones and teeth:

Micronutrients such as calcium, phosphorus, and vitamin D are important for maintaining strong bones and teeth, as well as preventing bone diseases such as osteoporosis.

Regulating metabolism:
Micronutrients such as B vitamins and minerals like magnesium and zinc are important for regulating metabolism and converting food into energy.

Supporting brain function:

Micronutrients such as omega-3 fatty acids and vitamins B6, B12, and folate are important for brain function, including memory, concentration, and mood regulation.

Preventing chronic diseases:

Micronutrients, such as antioxidants found in vitamins A, C, and E, and minerals such as selenium, can help prevent chronic diseases such as cancer, heart disease, and diabetes. It is important to ensure that you are getting adequate amounts of micronutrients in your diet to support overall health and well-being.

The DASH diet is rich in a variety of micronutrients, as it emphasizes whole, minimally processed foods that are naturally rich in vitamins and minerals.

However, it may be necessary to supplement with certain micronutrients, particularly for individuals with specific health conditions or dietary restrictions

How to create a balanced diet

Creating a balanced diet involves including a variety of foods from each food group in appropriate proportions to meet your individual nutritional needs.

Here are some general tips for creating a balanced diet:

Choose a variety of fruits and vegetables:

Aim to eat a variety of colorful fruits and vegetables each day, as they provide a range of essential vitamins, minerals, and fiber.

Include whole grains:
Choose whole grains such as brown rice, quinoa, whole wheat bread, and oatmeal over refined grains, as they provide more fiber and nutrients.

Incorporate lean protein sources:
Choose lean protein sources such as chicken, turkey, fish, beans, and nuts to provide the body with essential amino acids and other nutrients.

Include healthy fats:

Incorporate healthy fats such as those found in nuts, seeds, avocado, and olive oil, as they provide important nutrients and can help reduce inflammation and lower the risk of heart disease.

Limit processed and high-sugar foods:

Try to limit highly processed and high-sugar foods, as they provide empty calories and can contribute to weight gain and other health problems.

Stay hydrated:
Drink plenty of water throughout the day to help support digestion, hydration, and overall health.

It is also important to consider individual factors such as age, gender, activity level, and any specific health conditions or dietary restrictions when creating a balanced diet.

Consulting with a registered dietitian or healthcare provider can help ensure that your diet is tailored to your individual needs and goals

The impact of nutrition on health

Nutrition plays a crucial role in maintaining optimal health and preventing chronic diseases.

Here are some of the ways that nutrition impacts health

Energy and metabolism:
The food we eat provides the body with the energy and nutrients it needs to function properly. Adequate intake of macronutrients, such as carbohydrates, protein, and fat, is necessary to support the body's metabolism and energy needs.

Disease prevention:
A healthy diet that is rich in fruits, vegetables, whole grains, lean proteins, and healthy fats can help reduce the risk of chronic diseases such as heart disease, diabetes, and certain types of cancer.

Immune system function:

Adequate intake of micronutrients, such as vitamins A, C, and E, and zinc, is essential for proper immune system function and can help protect against infections and illnesses.

Brain function and mental health:

Proper nutrition is important for brain function and mental health.

A diet that is high in omega-3 fatty acids, vitamins, and antioxidants can help improve mood and cognitive function.

Bone health:

Adequate intake of calcium, vitamin D, and other nutrients is important for maintaining healthy bones and reducing the risk of osteoporosis and other bone-related diseases.

Weight management:

A healthy diet that is rich in whole, minimally processed foods can help promote healthy weight management and reduce the risk of obesity and related health problems.

Overall, nutrition plays a critical role in maintaining optimal health and preventing chronic diseases. Eating a balanced diet that is rich in a variety of nutrient-dense foods is key to achieving and maintaining good health.

CHAPTER THREE

MEAL PLANNING ON THE DASH DIET

How to plan meals on the DASH diet

Planning meals on the DASH diet involves incorporating a variety of nutrient-dense foods in appropriate portions to meet your individual dietary needs.

Here are some steps for meal planning on the DASH diet:

Determine your calorie needs:

Use an online calculator or work with a registered dietitian to determine your daily calorie needs based on your age, sex, height, weight, and activity level.

Divide your calories among macronutrients:

The DASH diet emphasizes a balance of macronutrients, with approximately 50% of calories coming from carbohydrates, 20-30% coming from protein, and 20-30% coming from healthy fats.

Choose foods from each food group:

The DASH diet emphasizes whole, minimally processed foods from all food groups, including fruits, vegetables, whole grains, lean proteins, and healthy fats.

Incorporate variety:

Aim to include a variety of foods from each food group throughout the day and week to provide the body with essential vitamins, minerals, and nutrients.

Plan ahead:

Use a meal planning tool or app to plan meals and snacks for the week ahead of time, taking into account your schedule, food preferences, and dietary needs.

Prep meals and snacks in advance:

Prepping meals and snacks in advance can help make healthy eating easier and more convenient. Try batch-cooking meals, chopping vegetables in advance, or packing snacks to bring with you on-the-go.

Use DASH diet-friendly recipes:
Incorporating DASH diet-friendly recipes into your meal plan can help ensure you are getting a variety of nutrient-dense foods and flavors.

Remember, meal planning on the DASH diet is not one-size-fits-all, and it may be helpful to work with a registered dietitian to develop a meal plan that meets your individual needs and preferences.

Tips for grocery shopping on the DASH diet

Grocery shopping on the DASH diet can be made easier by following these tips:

Make a list:

Before you go to the grocery store, make a list of the foods you need based on your meal plan for the week. This can help you stay on track and avoid impulse purchases.

Shop the perimeter of the store:
In general, the perimeter of the grocery store contains fresh, whole foods like fruits, vegetables, lean proteins, and dairy products, which are all DASH diet-friendly.

Choose fresh produce:

Aim to incorporate a variety of fresh fruits and vegetables into your diet. Choose in-season produce when possible, and look for pre-cut options to save time.

Read labels:

When purchasing packaged foods, read the nutrition labels to ensure they meet DASH diet guidelines. Look for products that are low in sodium and added sugars, and high in fiber.

Choose whole grains:

Choose whole-grain breads, cereals, and pastas, which are higher in fiber and other important nutrients than their refined counterparts.

Stock up on healthy fats:
Choose foods rich in healthy fats, such as nuts, seeds, avocado, and olive oil.

Look for lean proteins:

Choose lean protein sources, such as chicken, turkey, fish, beans, and tofu, which are lower in saturated fat and calories than some other protein sources.

Limit processed and high-sugar foods:

Avoid highly processed and high-sugar foods, as they can be high in calories and contribute to weight gain and other health problems.

Consider frozen and canned options:

Frozen and canned fruits and vegetables can be a convenient and cost-effective option, as long as they are low in sodium and added sugars.

By following these tips, you can make grocery shopping on the DASH diet easier and more efficient while still enjoying a variety of delicious and nutritious foods.

How to meal prep for the DASH diet

Meal prepping is an excellent way to save time and ensure that you have healthy, DASH diet-friendly meals available throughout the week.

Here are some tips for meal prepping on the DASH diet:

Plan your meals:

Before you start meal prepping, plan out your meals for the week. This can help you determine what ingredients you need and how much food to prepare.

Batch cook:

Choose one day of the week to batch cook several meals at once. You can make large batches of soups, stews, casseroles, or roasted vegetables that you can divide into individual portions and store in the fridge or freezer.

Portion control:

Use portion control containers or kitchen scales to ensure that you're eating the right amount of food. This can also help you manage your calorie intake.

Use glass containers:

Store your prepped meals in glass containers that are safe for the microwave and dishwasher. This can help you save time and minimize cleanup.

Keep it simple:

Choose simple recipes that are easy to prepare and require minimal ingredients. This can help you save time and minimize food waste.

Incorporate a variety of foods:

Choose a variety of fruits, vegetables, lean proteins, and whole grains to ensure that you're getting a well-rounded diet.

Pre-cut vegetables:

Pre-cut vegetables like carrots, celery, and cucumbers can be a great snack option throughout the week**Use healthy snacks:**

 Pre-portioned healthy snacks like nuts, seeds, and fruit can help keep you full between meals.

By following these tips, you can meal prep for the DASH diet and save time while still eating healthy, delicious meals

How to create balanced meals on the DASH diet

Creating balanced meals on the DASH diet can be done by following these simple steps:

Start with a base of whole grains:

Choose whole grains such as brown rice, quinoa, or whole-wheat pasta as the foundation of your meal. These grains are rich in fiber and provide essential vitamins and minerals.

Add vegetables:
Incorporate a variety of colorful vegetables into your meals. Choose leafy greens, peppers, carrots, broccoli, and other nutrient-rich vegetables.

Include lean protein:

Choose lean protein sources such as chicken, turkey, fish, tofu, beans, or lentils. These protein sources are lower in saturated fat and provide essential amino acids.

Use healthy fats:

Include healthy fats such as nuts, seeds, avocado, or olive oil in your meals. These fats provide essential fatty acids that help with brain function and reduce inflammation.

Season with herbs and spices:

Use herbs and spices to add flavor to your meals instead of salt. This can help reduce your sodium intake, which is a key component of the DASH diet.

Choose low-fat dairy:
If you include dairy in your meals, choose low-fat or non-fat options such as yogurt, milk, or cheese.

Incorporate fruits:
Add fruits to your meals as a healthy dessert or snack option. Choose a variety of fruits to ensure you are getting a range of vitamins and minerals.

By following these steps, you can create balanced and healthy meals on the DASH diet that provide all the essential nutrients your body needs to function properly.

CHAPTER FOUR

BREAKFAST RECIPES

Oatmeal recipes

Here are three oatmeal recipes that are DASH diet-friendly:

Apple Cinnamon Oatmeal:

Ingredients:

- 1 cup rolled oats

- 2 cups water

- 1/2 cup unsweetened applesauce

- 1/2 tsp cinnamon

- 1/4 tsp salt

- 1/4 cup chopped walnuts (optional)

Instructions:

- Combine oats, water, applesauce, cinnamon, and salt in a medium saucepan.

- Bring to a boil, then reduce heat and simmer for 5 minutes or until oats are tender and mixture has thickened.

- Serve hot, topped with chopped walnuts if desired.

Banana Nut Oatmeal:

Ingredients:

- 1 cup rolled oats

- 2 cups water

- 1 medium banana, mashed

- 1/4 cup chopped pecans

- 1/4 tsp cinnamon

- 1/4 tsp salt

Instructions:

- Combine oats, water, mashed banana, cinnamon, and salt in a medium saucepan.

- Bring to a boil, then reduce heat and simmer for 5 minutes or until oats are tender and mixture has thickened.

- Serve hot, topped with chopped pecans.

Blueberry Almond Oatmeal:
Ingredients:

- 1 cup rolled oats

- 2 cups water

- 1/2 cup blueberries (fresh or frozen)

- 2 tbsp sliced almonds

- 1/4 tsp vanilla extract

- 1/4 tsp salt

Instructions:

- Combine oats, water, blueberries, vanilla extract, and salt in a medium saucepan.

- Bring to a boil, then reduce heat and simmer for 5 minutes or until oats are tender and mixture has thickened.

- Serve hot, topped with sliced almonds.

These oatmeal recipes are not only delicious, but they are also packed with fiber and other nutrients that are essential for a healthy diet.

Smoothie recipes

Here are three DASH diet-friendly smoothie recipes:

Blueberry Spinach Smoothie:

Ingredients:

- 1 cup frozen blueberries

- 1/2 cup spinach leaves

- 1/2 cup unsweetened almond milk

- 1/2 cup plain Greek yogurt

- 1 tsp honey

Instructions:

- Combine all ingredients in a blender and blend until smooth.
- If the smoothie is too thick, add more almond milk as needed. Pour into a glass and enjoy!

Mango Banana Smoothie:

Ingredients:

- 1 cup frozen mango chunks
- 1 medium banana
- 1/2 cup unsweetened almond milk
- 1/2 cup plain Greek yogurt
- 1 tsp honey

Instructions:

- Combine all ingredients in a blender and blend until smooth.
- If the smoothie is too thick, add more almond milk as needed.,
- Pour into a glass and enjoy!

Green Apple Smoothie:

Ingredients:

- 1 medium green apple, chopped
- 1/2 cup spinach leaves

- 1/2 cup unsweetened almond milk

- 1/2 cup plain Greek yogurt

- 1 tsp honey

Instructions:

- Combine all ingredients in a blender and blend until smooth.

- If the smoothie is too thick, add more almond milk as needed.

- Pour into a glass and enjoy!

These smoothie recipes are quick, easy, and nutritious. They are a great way to get in some fruits and veggies in a tasty way.

Egg-based dishes

Here are three DASH diet-friendly egg-based dish recipes:

Veggie Omelet:

Ingredients:

- 2 eggs

- 1/4 cup chopped spinach

- 1/4 cup chopped tomatoes

- 1/4 cup chopped bell peppers

- 1/4 cup shredded cheddar cheese

- Salt and pepper to taste

- 1 tsp olive oil

Instructions:

- Whisk the eggs in a bowl and add salt and pepper to taste.

- Heat the olive oil in a non-stick pan over medium-high heat.
- Add the chopped veggies and sauté for 2-3 minutes until they are slightly softened.

- Pour the whisked eggs into the pan and cook for 2-3 minutes.

- Sprinkle the shredded cheese on one half of the omelet and fold the other half over the cheese.

- Cook for another 1-2 minutes until the cheese is melted and the eggs are cooked.

- Serve hot.

Egg and Veggie Muffins:

Ingredients:

- 6 eggs
- 1/2 cup chopped spinach
- 1/2 cup chopped tomatoes
- 1/2 cup chopped bell peppers
- Salt and pepper to taste

- Cooking spray

Instructions:
- Preheat the oven to 350°F (175°C).

- Whisk the eggs in a bowl and add salt and pepper to taste.

- Add the chopped veggies to the egg mixture and mix well.

- Spray a muffin tin with cooking spray.

- Pour the egg and veggie mixture into the muffin cups.

- Bake for 20-25 minutes until the eggs are cooked and golden brown.

- Remove from the oven and let cool for a few minutes.

- Remove the egg muffins from the muffin tin and serve.

Huevos Rancheros:

Ingredients:
- 2 eggs

- 1/2 cup black beans

- 1/4 cup chopped tomatoes

- 1/4 cup chopped onions

- 1/4 cup shredded cheddar cheese

- 1/4 cup salsa

- 2 whole wheat tortilla

- Salt and pepper to taste
- Cooking spray

Instructions:

- Spray a non-stick pan with cooking spray and heat over medium-high heat.

- Add the chopped onions and sauté for 2-3 minutes until they are slightly softened.

- Add the black beans and tomatoes to the pan and cook for another 2-3 minutes.

- In a separate pan, cook the eggs to your preference (scrambled, fried, or poached).

- Warm the tortillas in the microwave or oven.

- Place the tortillas on a plate and top with the black bean and veggie mixture.

- Add the cooked eggs on top of the bean mixture.

Sprinkle the shredded cheese over the eggs and top with salsa.

- Serve hot.

These egg-based dish recipes are high in protein, low in fat, and full of healthy veggies. They are perfect for a quick and easy breakfast, lunch, or dinner.

Healthy pancake and waffle recipes

Whole Wheat Banana Pancakes:

Ingredients:

- 1 cup whole wheat flour
- 1 tbsp baking powder
- 1/4 tsp salt
- 1 ripe banana, mashed
- 1 egg
- 1 cup nonfat milk
- 1 tbsp honey
- 1 tsp vanilla extract

Directions:

- In a bowl, mix together flour, baking powder, and salt.
- In another bowl, whisk together mashed banana, egg, milk, honey, and vanilla extract.
- Add the dry ingredients to the wet ingredients and mix until just combined.
- Heat a non-stick skillet over medium heat.
- Using a 1/4 cup measure, pour batter onto the skillet.

- Cook until bubbles form on the surface, then flip and cook until golden brown.
- Repeat with remaining batter.

Blueberry Oatmeal Pancakes:

Ingredients:

- 1 cup old-fashioned oats
- 1/2 cup whole wheat flour
- 1 tbsp baking powder
- 1/4 tsp salt
- 1/2 tsp cinnamon
- 1 egg
- 1 cup nonfat milk
- 1 tbsp honey
- 1 tsp vanilla extract
- 1 cup blueberries

Directions:

- In a bowl, mix together oats, flour, baking powder, salt, and cinnamon.
- In another bowl, whisk together egg, milk, honey, and vanilla extract.
- Add the dry ingredients to the wet ingredients and mix until just combined.

- Fold in blueberries.

- Heat a non-stick skillet over medium heat.

- Using a 1/4 cup measure, pour batter onto the skillet.

- Cook until bubbles form on the surface, then flip and cook until golden brown.

- Repeat with remaining batter.

Whole Wheat Banana Waffles:

Ingredients:

- 1 1/2 cups whole wheat flour

- 1 tbsp baking powder
- 1/4 tsp salt

- 1 ripe banana, mashed

- 2 eggs

- 1 cup nonfat milk

- 1 tbsp honey
- 1 tsp vanilla extract

Directions:

- In a bowl, mix together flour, baking powder, and salt.

- In another bowl, whisk together mashed banana, eggs, milk, honey, and vanilla extract.

- Add the dry ingredients to the wet ingredients and mix until just combined.

- Preheat a waffle iron according to manufacturer's instructions.
- Pour batter onto the waffle iron and cook until golden brown.
- Repeat with remaining batter.

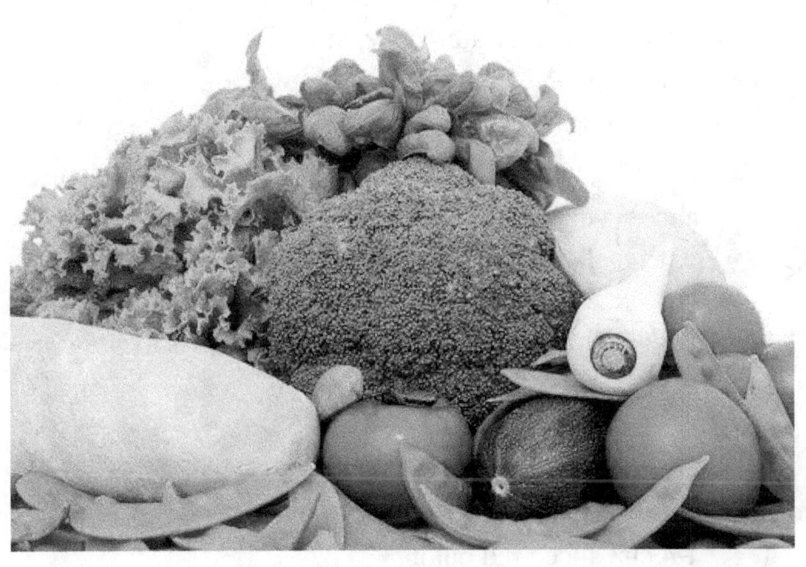

CHAPTER FIVE

LUNCH RECIPES

Salad recipes

Here are some salad recipes for the DASH diet:
- Spinach and Strawberry Salad:
- 2 cups baby spinach
- 1/2 cup sliced strawberries

- 1/4 cup chopped walnuts
- 1/4 cup crumbled feta cheese
- 1 tablespoon balsamic vinegar
- 1 tablespoon olive oil

Instructions:

- In a large bowl, add the spinach, strawberries, walnuts, and feta cheese.
- In a small bowl, whisk together the balsamic vinegar and olive oil.
- Drizzle the dressing over the salad and toss to combine.

Grilled Chicken Salad:
- 2 cups mixe greens
- 1/2 cup sliced cherry tomatoes
- 1/2 cup sliced cucumber
- 1/4 cup sliced red onion
- 4 oz grilled chicken breast
- 1 tablespoon red wine vinegar
- 1 tablespoon olive oil

Instructions:

- In a large bowl, add the mixed greens, cherry tomatoes, cucumber, and red onion.
- Slice the grilled chicken breast and add it to the salad.
- In a small bowl, whisk together the red wine vinegar and olive oil.
- Drizzle the dressing over the salad and toss to combine.

Tuna Salad:

- 2 cups mixed greens
- 1/4 cup sliced celery
- 1/4 cup sliced red onion
- 1 can tuna, drained
- 1 tablespoon lemon juice
- 1 tablespoon olive oil

Instructions:

- In a large bowl, add the mixed greens, celery, and red onion.
- Add the drained tuna to the bowl.
- In a small bowl, whisk together the lemon juice and olive oil.
- Drizzle the dressing over the salad and toss to combine.

Roasted Beet Salad:

- 2 cups mixed greens
- 1/4 cup sliced red onion
- 1/4 cup crumbled goat cheese

- 1/4 cup chopped walnuts
- 1 roasted beet, sliced
- 1 tablespoon red wine vinegar
- 1 tablespoon olive oil

Instructions:

- In a large bowl, add the mixed greens and red onion.
- Add the crumbled goat cheese and chopped walnuts to the bowl.
- Slice the roasted beet and add it to the salad.
- In a small bowl, whisk together the red wine vinegar and olive oil.
- Drizzle the dressing over the salad and toss to combine.

Soup recipes

Soup recipes for the DASH diet:

Vegetable Soup:

- 1 tablespoon olive oil
- 1 onion, diced
- 2 garlic cloves, minced
- 2 carrots, diced
- 2 celery stalks, diced
- 1 zucchini, diced
- 1 yellow squash, diced
- 1 can diced tomatoes
- 4 cups low-sodium vegetable broth
- 1 teaspoon dried oregano
- 1 teaspoon dried basil.
- Salt and pepper to taste

Instructions:

- Heat the olive oil in a large pot over medium heat.
- Add the onion and garlic and cook until softened, about 5 minutes.
- Add the carrots, celery, zucchini, and yellow squash and cook for another 5 minutes.
- Add the diced tomatoes, vegetable broth, oregano, basil, salt, and pepper.
- Bring the soup to a boil, then reduce the heat and let it simmer for 15-20 minutes.

Lentil Soup:

- 1 tablespoon olive oil
- 1 onion, diced
- 2 garlic cloves, minced
- 2 carrots, diced
- 2 celery stalks, diced
- 1 cup dry lentils
- 4 cups low-sodium vegetable broth
- 1 teaspoon ground cumin
- 1 teaspoon smoked paprika
- Salt and pepper to taste

Instructions:

- Heat the olive oil in a large pot over medium heat.
- Add the onion and garlic and cook until softened, about 5 minutes.
- Add the carrots and celery and cook for another 5 minutes.
- Add the lentils, vegetable broth, cumin, smoked paprika, salt, and pepper.

- Bring the soup to a boil, then reduce the heat and let it simmer for 30-40 minutes, or until the lentils are tender.
- Serve hot.

Chicken Noodle Soup:

- 1 tablespoon olive oil

- 1 onion, diced

- 2 garlic cloves, minced

- 2 carrots, diced

- 2 celery stalks, diced

- 4 cups low-sodium chicken broth

- 2 cups water

- 1 cup cooked chicken breast, shredded

- 1 cup whole wheat egg noodles

- 1 teaspoon dried thyme

- Salt and pepper to taste

Instructions:

- Heat the olive oil in a large pot over medium heat.

- Add the onion and garlic and cook until softened, about 5 minutes.

- Add the carrots and celery and cook for another 5 minutes.

- Add the chicken broth, water, cooked chicken breast, whole wheat egg noodles, thyme, salt, and pepper.

- Bring the soup to a boil, then reduce the heat and let it simmer for 10-15 minutes, or until the noodles are tender.

- Serve hot.

Sandwich recipes

Here are some sandwich recipes that you can try on the DASH diet:

Grilled Veggie and Hummus Sandwich:

- Whole grain bread

- Hummus

- Grilled zucchini, bell peppers, and onion

- Arugula

Tuna Salad Sandwich:

Whole grain bread

- Tuna canned in water, drained

- Greek yogurt

- Diced celery

- Diced red onion

- Salt and pepper to taste

Chicken and Avocado Sandwich:

- Whole grain bread
- Grilled chicken breast
- Avocado
- Tomato slices
- Lettuce
- Mustard

Veggie and Hummus Wrap:

- Whole wheat tortilla
- Hummus
- Shredded carrots
- Sliced cucumber
- Sliced bell pepper
- Arugula

Turkey and Cheese Sandwich:

- Whole grain bread
- Turkey breast slices
- Low-fat cheese
- Tomato slices
- Lettuce
- Mustard

Caprese Sandwich:

- Whole grain bread

- Fresh mozzarella

- Sliced tomato

- Fresh basil leaves

- Balsamic vinegar

Egg Salad Sandwich:

- Whole grain bread

- Hard-boiled eggs, chopped

- Greek yogurt

- Dijon mustard

- Chopped celery

- Salt and pepper to taste

- Lettuce

Buddha bowl recipes

Buddha bowls are a great way to create a balanced and healthy meal on the DASH diet.

Here are some Buddha bowl recipes to try:

Mediterranean Buddha Bowl:

* Quinoa

* Grilled chicken

* Cherry tomatoes

* Cucumber

* Kalamata olives

* Feta cheese

* Hummus

* Lemon wedges

Sweet Potato and Black Bean Buddha Bowl:

* Brown rice

* Roasted sweet potato

* Black beans

* Avocado

* Red onion

* Cilantro

* Lime wedges

* Greek yogurt

Asian Buddha Bowl:

* Brown rice

* Grilled salmon

* Steamed broccoli

- Carrots

- Edamame

- Cucumber

- Green onion

- Sesame seeds

- Soy sauce

Greek Quinoa Buddha Bowl:

- Quinoa

- Grilled chicken

- Cherry tomatoes

- Cucumber

- Red onion

- Kalamata olives

- Feta cheese

- Tzatziki sauce

Taco Buddha Bowl:

Brown rice

Ground turkey, cooked with taco seasoning

- Black beans

- Avocado

- Cherry tomatoes

- Red onion

- Cheddar cheese

- Salsa

- Greek yogurt

Roasted Vegetable Buddha Bowl:

- Quinoa

- Roasted sweet potato

- Roasted Brussels sprouts

- Roasted cauliflower

- Chickpeas

- Tahini dressing

Falafel Buddha Bowl:

- Quinoa

- Falafel balls

- Cherry tomatoes

- Cucumber

- Red onion

- Tzatziki sauce

- Hummus

Note: Adjust the ingredient quantities based on your individual needs and preferences, and make sure to choose whole grains, lean proteins, and plenty of vegetables for a balanced and nutritious Buddha bowl.

CHAPTER SIX
DINNER RECIPES

Roasted vegetable recipes

Roasted vegetables are a delicious and healthy addition to any meal on the DASH diet.

Here are some easy roasted vegetable recipes to try:

Roasted Brussels sprouts:

- Brussels sprouts
- Olive oil
- Salt and pepper
- Balsamic vinegar (optional)

Preheat oven to 400°F. Trim the ends of the Brussels sprouts and cut them in half. Toss with olive oil, salt, and pepper. Roast for 20-25 minutes, stirring once or twice, until tender and browned. Drizzle with balsamic vinegar before serving, if desired.

Roasted Sweet Potatoes:

- Sweet potatoes
- Olive oil
- Salt and pepper
- Cinnamon (optional)

Preheat oven to 400°F. Peel and cube the sweet potatoes. Toss with olive oil, salt, and pepper. Roast for 25-30 minutes, stirring once or twice, until tender and caramelized. Sprinkle with cinnamon before serving, if desired.

Roasted Cauliflower:

- Cauliflower
- Olive oil
- Salt and pepper
- Paprika (optional)

Preheat oven to 400°F. Cut the cauliflower into florets. Toss with olive oil, salt, and pepper. Roast for 25-30 minutes, stirring once or twice, until tender and golden. Sprinkle with paprika before serving, if desired.

Roasted Carrots:

- Carrots
- Olive oil
- Salt and pepper
- Honey (optional)

Preheat oven to 400°F. Peel and slice the carrots into rounds. Toss with olive oil, salt, and pepper. Roast for 20-

25 minutes, stirring once or twice, until tender and browned. Drizzle with honey before serving, if desired.

Roasted Broccoli:

- Broccoli
- Olive oil
- Salt and pepper
- Garlic (optional)

Preheat oven to 400°F. Cut the broccoli into florets. Toss with olive oil, salt, and pepper. Roast for 20-25 minutes, stirring once or twice, until tender and crispy. Add minced garlic halfway through roasting, if desired.

Note: Adjust the ingredient quantities and cooking time based on your individual needs and preferences. Roasted vegetables are a versatile and delicious addition to any meal, and can be enjoyed on their own or added to salads, grain bowls, or pasta dishes.

Lean protein recipes

Lean proteins are an essential part of a balanced diet, and there are many delicious and healthy options to choose from.

Here are some easy lean protein recipes to try on the DASH diet:

- Baked Salmon:
- Salmon fillets
- Lemon juice
- Olive oil
- Salt and pepper

Preheat oven to 375°F. Place salmon fillets on a baking sheet lined with parchment paper. Drizzle with lemon juice and olive oil, then sprinkle with salt and pepper. Bake for 12-15 minutes, or until cooked through and flaky.

Grilled Chicken:

- Chicken breasts
- Olive oil
- Salt and pepper
- Garlic powder (optional)

Preheat grill to medium-high heat. Brush chicken breasts with olive oil, then sprinkle with salt, pepper, and garlic powder. Grill for 6-8 minutes per side, or until cooked through and no longer pink.

Turkey Meatballs:

- Ground turkey

- Whole wheat breadcrumbs

- Egg

- Garlic powder

- Salt and pepper

- Marinara sauce

Preheat oven to 375°F. In a mixing bowl, combine ground turkey, whole wheat breadcrumbs, egg, garlic powder, salt, and pepper. Mix well, then shape into meatballs. Place meatballs on a baking sheet lined with parchment paper. Bake for 20-25 minutes, or until cooked through. Serve with marinara sauce.

Lentil Soup:

- Brown lentils
- Carrots
- Celery
- Onion
- Garlic

Low-sodium chicken broth

- Bay leaves
- Thyme
- Salt and pepper

In a large pot, sauté chopped carrots, celery, onion, and garlic in olive oil until tender. Add brown lentils, low-sodium chicken broth, bay leaves, thyme, salt, and pepper. Bring to a boil, then reduce heat and simmer for 30-35 minutes, or until lentils are tender. Serve hot.

Tuna Salad:

- Canned tuna
- Plain Greek yogurt
- Dijon mustard
- Lemon juice
- Salt and pepper

- Chopped celery
- Chopped red onion
- Chopped parsley

In a mixing bowl, combine canned tuna, plain Greek yogurt, Dijon mustard, lemon juice, salt, and pepper. Mix well, then add chopped celery, red onion, and parsley. Stir until well combined. Serve chilled.

Note: Adjust the ingredient quantities based on your individual needs and preferences. These lean protein recipes are easy to prepare and can be enjoyed as a main dish or as part of a larger meal.

Whole grain recipes

Here are some whole grain recipes that could be included in a DASH diet cookbook:

Quinoa and Black Bean Salad: Cook quinoa according to package directions and mix with canned black beans, chopped bell peppers, cherry tomatoes, red onion, cilantro, and a squeeze of fresh lime juice. Serve as a side dish or over a bed of lettuce for a satisfying meal.

Whole Wheat Pasta with Roasted

Vegetables: Roast your favorite vegetables (such as zucchini, eggplant, bell peppers, and onions) and toss with whole wheat pasta, a drizzle of olive oil, and some freshly grated Parmesan cheese.

Brown Rice Bowl with Veggies and Chicken:

Cook brown rice and serve in a bowl topped with grilled chicken, steamed vegetables (such as broccoli and carrots), and a drizzle of teriyaki sauce.

Barley and Lentil Soup:

Cook barley and lentils in vegetable broth with diced carrots, celery, onion, and garlic. Season with thyme and rosemary for a flavorful and filling soup.

Whole Grain Breakfast Bowl:

Cook steel-cut oats according to package directions and serve in a bowl topped with sliced banana, blueberries, chopped walnuts, and a drizzle of honey.

Whole Grain Veggie Wrap:

Spread hummus on a whole grain wrap and fill with sliced avocado, roasted red peppers, shredded carrots, and sliced cucumber.

Spicy Bulgur and Bean Salad:

Cook bulgur according to package directions and mix with canned black beans, diced tomatoes, chopped jalapeño peppers, red onion, and cilantro. Dress with a mixture of olive oil, lime juice, and cumin for a flavorful and spicy salad.

Whole Grain Pizza:

Use a whole grain pizza crust and top with your favorite veggies and lean protein (such as chicken or turkey sausage) for a healthier version of pizza.

Quinoa Stuffed Peppers:

Cook quinoa and mix with diced tomatoes, black beans, corn, and cilantro. Stuff the mixture into halved bell peppers and bake until tender.

Whole Grain Muffins:

Bake muffins with whole grain flour and add in fruits and nuts for added nutrition and flavor.

One-pot meal recipes

Here are some one-pot meal recipes that could be included in a DASH diet cookbook:

Chicken and Vegetable Stir Fry:

Cook chicken breast in a large skillet or wok with a small amount of oil until browned. Add chopped vegetables (such as bell peppers, broccoli, and carrots) and stir fry until tender. Serve over brown rice or quinoa.

Lentil and Vegetable Stew:

Cook lentils in vegetable broth with diced tomatoes, chopped carrots, celery, onion, and garlic. Season with thyme and rosemary for a flavorful and filling stew.

One-Pot Chicken and Brown Rice:
Cook chicken breast in a large pot with a small amount of oil until browned. Add brown rice, diced tomatoes, chicken broth, and a selection of vegetables (such as chopped zucchini and bell peppers) and bring to a simmer. Cover and cook until the rice is tender and the chicken is cooked through.

Shrimp and Veggie Skillet:
Cook shrimp in a large skillet with a small amount of oil until pink. Add sliced zucchini, diced tomatoes, chopped onion, and garlic and sauté until tender. Season with paprika and chili powder for a spicy kick.

Sausage and Lentil One-Pot:
Cook sausage in a large pot with a small amount of oil until browned. Add lentils, diced tomatoes, chicken broth, and chopped vegetables (such as carrots and celery) and bring to a simmer. Cover and cook until the lentils are tender and the sausage is cooked through.

Vegetable and Chickpea Curry:

Cook diced onion, garlic, and ginger in a large pot with a small amount of oil until softened. Add chopped vegetables (such as cauliflower and bell peppers) and canned chickpeas, along with curry powder and coconut milk. Simmer until the vegetables are tender and the sauce is thickened.

Quinoa and Vegetable Skillet:

Cook quinoa according to package directions and set aside. In a large skillet, cook chopped onion, bell pepper, zucchini, and garlic in a small amount of oil until tender. Stir in the cooked quinoa, diced tomatoes, and a selection of spices (such as cumin and chili powder) for a flavorful and filling one-pot meal.

Turkey and Sweet Potato Chili:

Cook ground turkey in a large pot with a small amount of oil until browned. Add diced sweet potato, canned diced tomatoes, black beans, and chili powder. Simmer until the sweet potato is tender and the chili is heated through.

Pasta with Veggies and White Beans:

Cook pasta according to package directions and set aside. In a large skillet, cook diced onion and garlic in a small amount of oil until softened. Add sliced bell pepper and chopped kale, along with canned white beans and diced tomatoes. Stir in the cooked pasta and season with a selection of herbs (such as basil and oregano).

One-Pot Mediterranean Chicken and Rice:

Cook chicken breast in a large pot with a small amount of oil until browned. Add brown rice, chopped vegetables (such as zucchini and red onion), diced tomatoes, chicken broth, and a selection of herbs (such as thyme and rosemary). Simmer until the rice is tender and the chicken is cooked through.

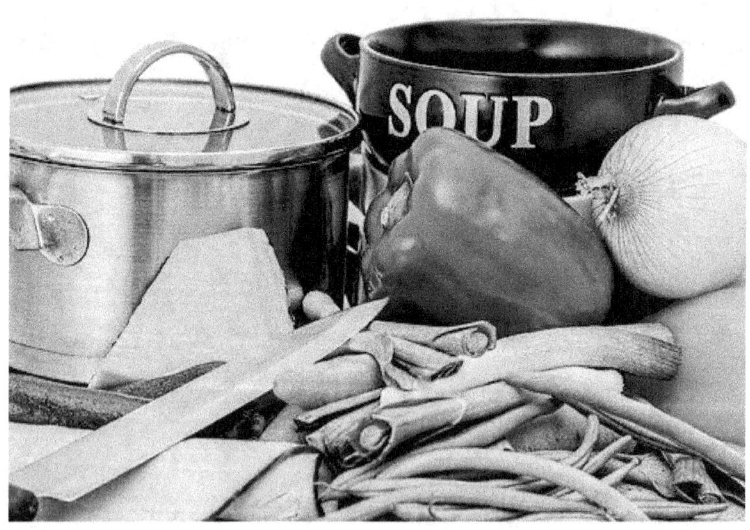

CHAPTER SEVEN

SNACK RECIPES

Fruit and nut bar recipes

These are some fruits and nut bar recipes that would be great for the DASH diet:

Blueberry Almond Bars

- 2 cups old-fashioned rolled oats

- 1 cup almonds, chopped

- 1/2 cup dried blueberries

- 1/4 cup honey

- 1/4 cup almond butter

- 1/4 cup coconut oil, melted

- 1 tsp vanilla extract

- 1/4 tsp salt

Directions:

- Preheat oven to 350°F. Line an 8-inch square baking pan with parchment paper.

- In a large bowl, mix together oats, almonds, and dried blueberries.

- In a small bowl, whisk together honey, almond butter, coconut oil, vanilla extract, and salt. Pour over oat mixture and stir until well combined.

- Press mixture into prepared pan and bake for 20-25 minutes or until golden brown. Let cool completely before cutting into bars.

Cherry Walnut Bars

- 2 cups old-fashioned rolled oats

- 1 cup walnuts, chopped

- 1/2 cup dried cherries

- 1/4 cup honey

- 1/4 cup almond butter

- 1/4 cup coconut oil, melted

- 1 tsp vanilla extract

- 1/4 tsp salt

Directions:

- Preheat oven to 350°F. Line an 8-inch square baking pan with parchment paper.

- In a large bowl, mix together oats, walnuts, and dried cherries.In a small bowl, whisk together honey, almond butter, coconut oil, vanilla extract, and salt. Pour over oat mixture and stir until well combined.

- Press mixture into prepared pan and bake for 20-25 minutes or until golden brown. Let cool completely before cutting into bars.

Apple Cinnamon Bars

- 2 cups old-fashioned rolled oats

- 1 cup pecans, chopped

- 1/2 cup dried apples, chopped

- 1/4 cup honey

- 1/4 cup almond butter

- 1/4 cup coconut oil, melted

- 1 tsp cinnamon

- 1/4 tsp salt

Directions:

- Preheat oven to 350°F. Line an 8-inch square baking pan with parchment paper.

- In a large bowl, mix together oats, pecans, and dried apples.

- In a small bowl, whisk together honey, almond butter, coconut oil, cinnamon, and salt. Pour over oat mixture and stir until well combined.

- Press mixture into prepared pan and bake for 20-25 minutes or until golden brown. Let cool completely before cutting into bars.

Vegetable dip recipes

Here are a few vegetable dip recipes for the DASH diet:

Hummus Dip

- 1 can chickpeas, drained and rinsed

- 2 cloves garlic, minced

- 2 tablespoons tahini

- 2 tablespoons lemon juice

- 2 tablespoons water

- 1 tablespoon olive oil

- Salt and pepper to taste

Instructions: In a food processor, combine all the ingredients and process until smooth. Serve with sliced vegetables.

Avocado Dip

- 2 ripe avocados, pitted and peeled
- 1/4 cup plain Greek yogurt
- 1 clove garlic, minced
- 1 tablespoon lime juice
- Salt and pepper to taste

Instructions: In a medium bowl, mash the avocado with a fork or potato masher. Stir in the Greek yogurt, garlic, and lime juice. Season with salt and pepper to taste. Serve with sliced vegetables.

Greek Yogurt Dip

- 1 cup plain Greek yogurt
- 1/2 cucumber, peeled and grated
- 2 cloves garlic, minced
- 1 tablespoon lemon juice
- 1 tablespoon chopped fresh dill
- Salt and pepper to taste

Instructions: In a medium bowl, stir together the Greek yogurt, grated cucumber, garlic, lemon juice, and dill. Season with salt and pepper to taste. Serve with sliced vegetables.

Black Bean Dip

- 1 can black beans, drained and rinsed
- 1/4 cup salsa
- 1/4 cup plain Greek yogurt
- 1 clove garlic, minced
- 1/2 teaspoon cumin
- Salt and pepper to taste

Instructions: In a food processor, combine the black beans, salsa, Greek yogurt, garlic, and cumin. Process until smooth. Season with salt and pepper to taste. Serve with sliced vegetables.

Smoothie recipes

Here are some smoothie recipes that can be incorporated into the DASH diet:

Berry Blast Smoothie:

- 1 cup mixed berries (strawberries, raspberries, blueberries)
- 1 banana
- 1/2 cup plain Greek yogurt
- 1/2 cup unsweetened almond milk
- 1 tablespoon honey

- Blend all ingredients together in a blender until smooth. Serve immediately.

Green Goddess Smoothie:

- 1 cup kale
- 1/2 cucumber
- 1/2 avocado
- 1/2 banana
- 1/2 cup unsweetened almond milk
- 1 tablespoon honey

Blend all ingredients together in a blender until smooth. Serve immediately.

Tropical Paradise Smoothie:

- 1/2 cup pineapple chunks
- 1/2 cup mango chunks
- 1/2 banana
- 1/2 cup plain Greek yogurt
- 1/2 cup unsweetened coconut milk

Blend all ingredients together in a blender until smooth. Serve immediately.

Peanut Butter Banana Smoothie:

- 1 banana
- 1 tablespoon natural peanut butter

- 1/2 cup plain Greek yogurt

- 1/2 cup unsweetened almond milk

- 1 teaspoon honey

Blend all ingredients together in a blender until smooth. Serve immediately.

Roasted chickpea recipes

Roasted chickpeas are a delicious and nutritious snack that can be enjoyed on the DASH diet. Here are some recipes to try:

Spicy Roasted Chickpeas:

- 1 can chickpeas, drained and rinsed

- 1 tablespoon olive oil

- 1/2 teaspoon cumin

- 1/2 teaspoon paprika

- 1/4 teaspoon cayenne pepper

- Salt and pepper to taste

Preheat oven to 400°F (200°C). In a bowl, toss the chickpeas with olive oil, cumin, paprika, cayenne pepper, salt, and pepper. Spread the chickpeas on a baking sheet in a single layer. Bake for 20-25 minutes, or until the chickpeas are crispy.

Sweet and Spicy Roasted Chickpeas:

- 1 can chickpeas, drained and rinsed
- 1 tablespoon olive oil
- 1 tablespoon honey
- 1/2 teaspoon chili powder
- Salt and pepper to taste

Preheat oven to 400°F (200°C). In a bowl, toss the chickpeas with olive oil, honey, chili powder, salt, and pepper. Spread the chickpeas on a baking sheet in a single layer. Bake for 20-25 minutes, or until the chickpeas are crispy.

Lemon and Herb Roasted Chickpeas:

- 1 can chickpeas, drained and rinsed
- 1 tablespoon olive oil
- 1 tablespoon lemon juice
- 1 teaspoon dried oregano
- 1 teaspoon dried thyme
- Salt and pepper to taste

Preheat oven to 400°F (200°C). In a bowl, toss the chickpeas with olive oil, lemon juice, oregano, thyme, salt, and pepper. Spread the chickpeas on a baking sheet in a single layer. Bake for 20-25 minutes, or until the chickpeas are crispy

Garlic and Parmesan Roasted Chickpeas:

1 can chickpeas, drained and rinsed

1 tablespoon olive oil

2 cloves garlic, minced

1/4 cup grated Parmesan cheese

Salt and pepper to taste

Preheat oven to 400°F (200°C). In a bowl, toss the chickpeas with olive oil, garlic, Parmesan cheese, salt, and pepper. Spread the chickpeas on a baking sheet in a single layer. Bake for 20-25 minutes, or until the chickpeas are crispy.

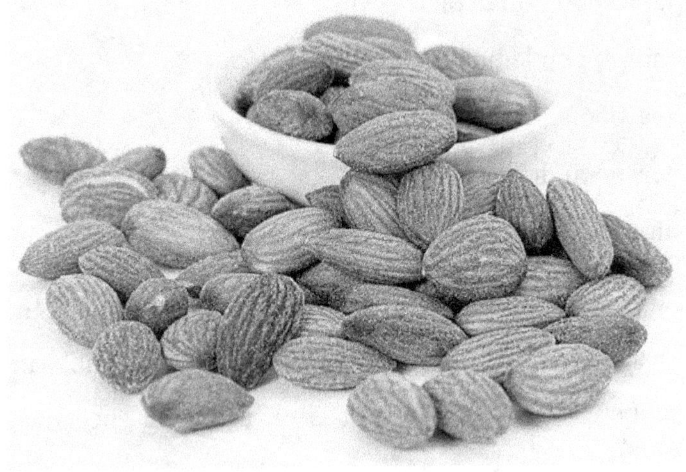

CHAPTER EIGHT
DESSERT RECIPES

Fruit crisp recipes

Apple Crisp

- 6 cups peeled and sliced apples
- ½ cup all-purpose flour
- ½ cup rolled oats
- ½ cup brown sugar
- ½ teaspoon cinnamon
- ½ cup unsalted butter, softened

Preheat oven to 375°F. Place sliced apples in a 9-inch baking dish. In a medium bowl, mix flour, oats, brown sugar, cinnamon, and butter until crumbly. Sprinkle mixture over apples. Bake for 45-50 minutes until apples are tender and the topping is golden brown.

Peach Crisp

- 4 cups sliced peaches
- ¼ cup all-purpose flour
- ¼ cup rolled oats
- ¼ cup brown sugar
- ½ teaspoon cinnamon

¼ cup unsalted butter, softened

Preheat oven to 375°F. Place sliced peaches in a 9-inch baking dish. In a medium bowl, mix flour, oats, brown sugar, cinnamon, and butter until crumbly. Sprinkle mixture over peaches. Bake for 35-40 minutes until peaches are tender and the topping is golden brown.

Mixed Berry Crisp

- 4 cups mixed berries (strawberries, blueberries, raspberries)
- ½ cup all-purpose flour
- ½ cup rolled oats
- ½ cup brown sugar
- ½ teaspoon cinnamon
- ½ cup unsalted butter, softened

Preheat oven to 375°F. Place mixed berries in a 9-inch baking dish. In a medium bowl, mix flour, oats, brown sugar, cinnamon, and butter until crumbly. Sprinkle mixture over berries. Bake for 35-40 minutes until berries are tender and the topping is golden brown.

Yogurt parfait recipes

Berry Yogurt Parfait:

- 1 cup plain Greek yogurt

- ½ cup mixed berries (such as strawberries, blueberries, and raspberries)

- ¼ cup granola

- 1 tablespoon honey

Layer the yogurt, berries, and granola in a bowl or jar. Drizzle with honey and serve.

- **Tropical Yogurt Parfait:**

- 1 cup plain Greek yogurt

- ½ cup chopped mango

- ½ cup chopped pineapple

- ¼ cup shredded coconut

Layer the yogurt, mango, pineapple, and coconut in a bowl or jar. Serve chilled.

Peanut Butter and Banana Yogurt Parfait:

- 1 cup plain Greek yogurt

- 1 banana, sliced

- 2 tablespoons natural peanut butter

- 2 tablespoons chopped peanuts

Layer the yogurt and banana in a bowl or jar. Drizzle with peanut butter and sprinkle with chopped peanuts. Serve chilled.

Chocolate Yogurt Parfait:

- 1 cup plain Greek yogurt
- ¼ cup unsweetened cocoa powder
- 2 tablespoons honey
- ¼ cup granola

Mix the yogurt, cocoa powder, and honey in a bowl. Layer the yogurt mixture and granola in a bowl or jar. Serve chilled.

Apple Cinnamon Yogurt Parfait:

- 1 cup plain Greek yogurt
- ½ cup chopped apple
- ¼ cup granola
- 1 teaspoon cinnamon

Layer the yogurt, apple, granola, and cinnamon in a bowl or jar. Serve chilled.

Low-sugar baked good recipes

Here are some low-sugar baked good recipes that you can try:

Low-Sugar Banana Bread:

Ingredients: 2 ripe bananas, mashed; 2 eggs; 1/3 cup melted coconut oil; ¼ cup unsweetened almond milk; 1 tsp vanilla extract; 2 cups almond flour; 2 tsp baking powder; ½ tsp baking soda; ¼ tsp salt.

Instructions: Preheat oven to 350°F. In a large mixing bowl, whisk together the mashed bananas, eggs, melted coconut oil, almond milk, and vanilla extract until well combined. In another bowl, mix together the almond flour, baking powder, baking soda, and salt. Add the dry ingredients to the wet ingredients and mix until well combined. Pour the batter into a greased loaf pan and bake for 50-60 minutes or until a toothpick inserted into the center comes out clean.

Low-Sugar Blueberry Muffins:

Ingredients: 2 cups almond flour; ¼ cup coconut flour; ¼ cup erythritol; 1 tsp baking powder; ½ tsp baking soda; ½ tsp salt; 3 eggs; ½ cup unsweetened almond milk; ¼ cup melted coconut oil; 1 tsp vanilla extract; 1 cup blueberries.

Instructions: Preheat oven to 350°F. In a large mixing bowl, mix together the almond flour, coconut flour, erythritol, baking powder, baking soda, and salt. In another bowl, whisk together the eggs, almond milk, melted coconut oil, and vanilla extract. Add the wet ingredients to the dry ingredients and mix until well combined. Fold in the blueberries. Pour the batter into greased muffin cups and bake for 20-25 minutes or until a toothpick inserted into the center comes out clean.

Low-Sugar Chocolate Chip Cookies:

Ingredients: 2 cups almond flour; ¼ cup coconut flour; ¼ cup erythritol; 1 tsp baking soda; ¼ tsp salt; ¼ cup melted coconut oil; ¼ cup almond butter; 2 eggs; 1 tsp vanilla extract; ½ cup sugar-free chocolate chips.

Instructions: Preheat oven to 350°F. In a large mixing bowl, mix together the almond flour, coconut flour, erythritol, baking soda, and salt. In another bowl, whisk together the melted coconut oil, almond butter, eggs, and vanilla extract. Add the wet ingredients to the dry ingredients and mix until well combined. Fold in the chocolate chips. Roll the dough into balls and place on a greased baking sheet. Bake for 10-12 minutes or until golden brown.

Pudding recipes

These are some healthy and delicious pudding recipes for the DASH diet:

Chia Seed Pudding:

- ½ cup chia seeds
- 2 cups almond milk
- ½ tsp vanilla extract
- 1 tbsp honey or maple syrup
- Fresh berries for topping

Instructions:

Mix chia seeds, almond milk, vanilla extract and honey/maple syrup in a bowl. Whisk until combined. Cover and refrigerate for at least 2 hours or overnight. Serve with fresh berries on top.

Banana Chocolate Pudding:

- 2 ripe bananas
- ½ cup unsweetened cocoa powder
- ¼ cup honey or maple syrup
- ¼ cup almond milk

- ½ tsp vanilla extract

Instructions:

Blend all ingredients in a blender until smooth. Pour into individual cups and refrigerate for at least 2 hours. Serve chilled.

Avocado Pudding:

- 2 ripe avocados
- ¼ cup unsweetened cocoa powder
- ¼ cup honey or maple syrup
- ¼ cup almond milk
- ½ tsp vanilla extract

Instructions:

Blend all ingredients in a blender until smooth. Pour into individual cups and refrigerate for at least 2 hours. Serve chilled.

Tapioca Pudding:

- ½ cup tapioca pearls
- 3 cups almond milk
- ¼ cup honey or maple syrup
- ½ tsp vanilla extract
- Fresh fruit for topping

Instructions:

Soak tapioca pearls in water for 30 minutes. Drain and rinse. In a pot, combine almond milk, tapioca pearls, honey/maple syrup and vanilla extract. Bring to a boil and simmer for 20-25 minutes, stirring frequently, until tapioca pearls are translucent. Let cool and refrigerate for at least 2 hours. Serve with fresh fruit on top.

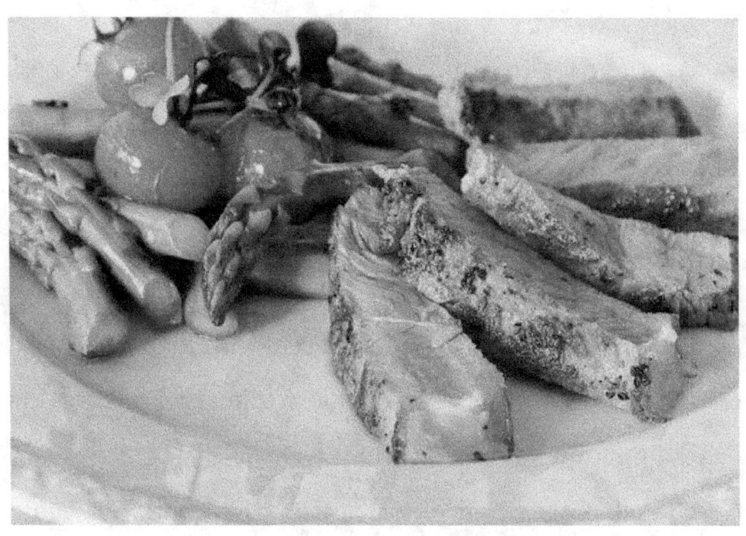

CHAPTER NINE

DASH DIET TIPS AND TRICKS

Eating out on the DASH diet

Eating out on the DASH diet can be challenging, but it's not impossible. With a little planning and knowledge, you can enjoy a meal out while still following the principles of the DASH diet.

Here are some tips for eating out on the DASH diet:

Choose wisely:

When you're looking at a menu, look for items that are high in vegetables, whole grains, and lean protein. Avoid items that are high in saturated fat, sodium, and added sugars.

Ask questions:

Don't be afraid to ask your server about how a dish is prepared or if certain ingredients can be substituted. Most restaurants are happy to accommodate dietary needs.

Watch portion sizes:

Restaurant portions are often larger than what you would serve at home. Consider sharing an entrée or taking half home for later.

Skip the extras:

Ask for dressings, sauces, and condiments on the side, and use them sparingly. Skip the breadbasket or ask for whole-grain bread instead of white.

Choose water or unsweetened beverages:

Sweetened drinks can add a lot of calories and sugar to your meal. Stick with water, unsweetened tea, or other low-calorie, low-sugar options.

Don't be afraid to customize:

If a menu item isn't quite right for you, don't be afraid to ask for substitutions or modifications. For example, you could ask for a side of steamed vegetables instead of fries.

Remember, eating out should be enjoyable. Don't stress too much about following the DASH diet perfectly while dining out – just do the best you can and enjoy your meal.

Staying on track while traveling

Maintaining a healthy diet while traveling can be challenging, but it is possible to stay on track with the DASH diet with some planning and preparation.

Here are some tips:

Research restaurants in advance:

Before you travel, research restaurants in the area and look for ones that offer healthy options or accommodate dietary restrictions.

Pack healthy snacks:

Pack healthy snacks such as fruit, nuts, and whole grain crackers to have on hand when you are traveling. This will help prevent you from making unhealthy food choices out of hunger.

Bring your own food:

If possible, bring your own food with you when traveling. This could include sandwiches, salads, or other healthy options that you can prepare in advance.

Choose wisely at restaurants:

When eating out, choose dishes that are grilled, baked, or broiled rather than fried. Ask for dressings and sauces on the side, and choose vegetables or salads as a side dish instead of fries.

Avoid sugary drinks:

Sugary drinks can add a lot of calories to your diet, so opt for water, unsweetened tea, or sparkling water instead.

Be mindful of portion sizes:

Pay attention to portion sizes when eating out, and try to avoid overeating. Ask for a to-go container and save half of your meal for later.

Stay active:

Staying active while traveling can help you burn calories and maintain a healthy weight. Look for opportunities to walk or bike, and consider packing a resistance band for a quick workout in your hotel room.

By following these tips, you can stay on track with the DASH diet while traveling and maintain a healthy lifestyle.

Snack ideas for the DASH diet

These are some snack ideas for the DASH diet:

- Greek yogurt with berries
- Apple slices with almond butter
- Carrot sticks with hummus
- Air-popped popcorn
- Edamame
- Mixed nuts and seeds
- Roasted chickpeas
- Cottage cheese with pineapple

- Avocado on whole grain toast

- Rice cakes with almond butter and banana slices

- Low-sodium turkey or ham slices with cucumber

- Hard-boiled eggs

- Fruit salad with a dollop of Greek yogurt

- Cheese stick with grapes

- Trail mix with dried fruit and nuts.

How to handle social situations on the DASH diet

Handling social situations while following the DASH diet can be challenging, but it is not impossible.

Here are some tips to help you navigate social situations while on the DASH diet:

Plan ahead:

If you know you will be attending a social event, try to plan ahead and research the menu or ask the host what food will be served. This way, you can plan your meals and snacks accordingly.

Bring your own dish:

Offer to bring a dish to the event that fits within the DASH diet guidelines. This way, you can ensure that you have a healthy option to eat.

Be mindful of portions:

If you cannot control what food is served, be mindful of portion sizes. Try to fill your plate with mostly fruits, vegetables, and lean protein sources.

Choose wisely:

When making food choices, opt for foods that are low in sodium and high in fiber. Avoid fried or processed foods and opt for grilled or baked options.

Drink plenty of water:

Drinking plenty of water can help you feel full and avoid overeating. Avoid sugary drinks and alcohol, which can be high in calories and sugar.

Focus on socializing:

Remember that social events are about spending time with friends and family, not just the food. Focus on the people and the conversation, rather than solely on the food.

CHAPTER TEN
CONCLUSION

Key takeaways from the book

Some possible key takeaways from "The DASH Diet Cookbook: Delicious, Easy, and Healthy Recipes to Lower Blood Pressure" could include:

The DASH diet is a healthy eating plan designed to help lower blood pressure and reduce the risk of heart disease, stroke, and other health problems.

The DASH diet emphasizes whole, unprocessed foods, including fruits, vegetables, whole grains, lean proteins, and low-fat dairy products.

Micronutrients such as vitamins and minerals play an important role in overall health, and the DASH diet can help ensure that you get enough of these essential nutrients. Meal planning and preparation are key to following the DASH diet and making healthy eating a habit.

The book provides a wide variety of delicious and easy recipes that are compliant with the DASH diet, including oatmeal, smoothies, egg dishes, salads, soups, sandwiches, Buddha bowls, roasted vegetables, lean proteins, whole grains, one-pot meals, fruit and nut bars, vegetable dips, low-sugar baked goods, and puddings.

The book also provides guidance on eating out and handling social situations while following the DASH diet. Overall, following the DASH diet and incorporating its principles into your everyday life can lead to improved health, lower blood pressure, and a reduced risk of chronic disease.

Encouragement to continue following the DASH diet

If you've made it this far and are considering following the DASH diet, congratulations! Choosing to prioritize your health and well-being is a big step. Remember that following a healthy diet is not about being perfect, but about making small, sustainable changes over time.

While it may be challenging at first, staying consistent with the DASH diet can bring about many positive changes in your health, including lower blood pressure, improved cholesterol levels, and decreased risk of chronic diseases such as heart disease and stroke. Keep in mind that these benefits can take time to manifest, so don't get discouraged if you don't see results right away.

Surround yourself with supportive friends and family members who will encourage you on your journey. Seek out resources such as cookbooks, online communities, and support groups to help you stay motivated and inspired.

Remember to be kind to yourself, and don't beat yourself up if you slip up or have a less-than-perfect day. Each day is a new opportunity to make healthy choices and take care of your body. With time and consistency, following the DASH diet can become a natural and enjoyable part of your daily life.

Additional resources for learning more about the DASH diet

Here are some additional resources for learning more about the DASH diet:

- National Heart, Lung, and Blood Institute (NHLBI) - The NHLBI provides extensive information on the DASH diet, including meal plans, recipes, and tips for following the diet. They also offer a free PDF version of "Your Guide to Lowering Your Blood Pressure with DASH."

- Mayo Clinic - The Mayo Clinic offers a comprehensive overview of the DASH diet, including its principles, health benefits, and recommended food groups. They also provide sample meal plans and recipes.

- DASH for Health - DASH for Health is an online program that provides personalized meal plans, recipes, and resources for following the DASH diet. They offer a 14-day free trial, and then charge a monthly fee for continued access to their resources.

- American Heart Association - The American Heart Association offers information on the DASH diet, as well as other dietary guidelines for maintaining heart health. They also provide recipes and meal planning resources.